Contents

What Is Hemochromatosis 7

What are the symptoms of hemochromatosis? ..8

What causes hemochromatosis? 10

How is hemochromatosis diagnosed? 12

How is hemochromatosis treated? 13

Who is at risk for hemochromatosis?.............15

What is the outlook with hemochromatosis?....16

Questions to Ask Your Doctor......................17

Hemochromatosis diet...............................18

Dietary factors 19

What to eat 21

What to avoid 25

HEMOCHROMATOSIS DIET RECIPES 30

Buttermilk Green Tea Roasted Roasted Chicken 30

Blueberry Salad with Grilled Tumeric Chicken..33

Vegetable Quiche 35

Turkey Chili 38

Argentine Diet Merenguitos..............................40

Glady Chicken veggie mix.................................43

Mac and Cheese in Power Pressure Cooker 45

Gradly Black Beans and Rice 47

Macaroni, Cheese and Broccoli Quesadilla.......48

Gradly Banana But Muffins (With Almond Milk) 51

Sixty's Vanilla Trivia Iced Decaf Coffee...........52

Gradly Pesto Pasta..53

Gradly Roasted Tomatoes and Broccoli Pasta ..55

Gladly Green Curry w/Turkey 57

Slow Cooker BBQ Shredded Pork Loin 59

Gradly Vanilla Ice cream.................................62

Overnight Vanilla Almond Chia Seed Pudding ..64

Gradly Spinach Enchiladas 66

Gradly Vegetable Coconut Rice.....................68

Overnight Chia Flax Pudding with Cherries......70

Gradly Low Fat Vanilla Ice cream..................71

Gradly Quickly Pasta 73

Pumpkin Kodiak Waffle.................................75

Gradly Creamy Grits 78

Mexican Shrimp Cocktail 81

Gradly's Mexi-call Chicken 84

Gradly Orange Chicken Teriyaki Rice...........86

Gradly Fruit Topping 87

Easy Granola 88

Marta Stewart's Chocolate Custard Cup 91

Chocolate Custard 94

Fudge Brownies/ Whole wheat 96

Quick Lentil Sauce and Spaghetti...................98

Baked Potato Flake and Fried Chicken Thighs 100

Quick Cheesy Salmon Noodle Bake 102

Maid Rites 105

Coachmn's Salad 106

Salad Ingredients (Cut in size of match sticks).

....107

Oatmeal, Oatbran, Flax 109

Kidney Bean and Taraggon Salad 110

Salmon Burger on a Bed of Baby Green........112

Stuffed Cabbage...115

Dilled Carrot, Cabbage and Parsnip Soup 118

Grated Raw Beet Salad 121

Tomatoes Avocado Relish (Salsa) 123

Eggplant Stacks 125

What Is Hemochromatosis

Hemochromatosis an inherited condition in which the body absorbs and stores too much iron. The extra iron builds up in several organs, especially the liver, and can cause serious damage. Without treatment, the disease can cause these organs to fail.

Iron is an essential nutrient found in many foods. Healthy people usually absorb about 10 percent of the iron contained in the food they eat to meet the body's needs.

People with hemochromatosis absorb more than the body needs. The body has no natural way to rid itself of the excess iron, causing the excess to build up in the organs.

What are the symptoms of hemochromatosis?

Many people have no symptoms, even in advanced cases. Joint pain is the most common complaint of people with hemochromatosis. Other common symptoms include

• Fatigue (feeling tired a lot).

• General weakness.

• Heart flutters or irregular heartbeat.

• "Iron fist," or pain in the knuckles of the pointer and middle fingers.

• Joint pain.

• Stomach pain.

• Unexplained weight loss.

• loss of sex drive.

Symptoms tend to occur in men between the ages of 30 and 50 and in women over age 50. However, many people have no symptoms when they are diagnosed.

If the disease is not detected early and treated, iron may accumulate in body tissues and may eventually lead to serious problems such as:

• arthritis

• liver disease, including an enlarged liver, cirrhosis, cancer, and liver failure

• damage to the pancreas, possibly causing diabetes

- heart abnormalities, such as irregular heart rhythms or congestive heart failure

- impotence

- early menopause

- abnormal pigmentation of the skin, making it look gray or bronze

- pituitary damage

- damage to the adrenal gland

What causes hemochromatosis?

Genetic or hereditary hemochromatosis is connected to a defect in a gene called HFE, which regulates the amount of iron absorbed from food.

While hemochromatosis is present at birth, symptoms rarely appear before adulthood. A person who inherits the defective gene from both parents may develop hemochromatosis. A person who inherits the defective gene from only one parent is a carrier for the disease but usually does not develop it.

Juvenile hemochromatosis and neonatal hemochromatosis are two forms of the disease that are not caused by a HFE defect. Their cause is unknown. The juvenile form leads to severe iron overload and liver and heart disease in adolescents and young adults between the ages of 15 and 30, and the neonatal form causes the same problems in newborn infants.

How is hemochromatosis diagnosed?

Blood tests for serum iron and either total iron binding capacity or transferrin are good screening tests. A good additional test is serum ferritin level, which is elevated in patients with hemochromatosis. If these tests are persistently high, a genetic test for the mutations in the HFE gene should be performed.

Depending on whether there is evidence of liver damage, a liver biopsy should be done to assess the damage to the liver. Excess iron is also frequently present in patients with alcoholic liver disease or chronic viral hepatitis. A liver biopsy is the only definitive way to determine if patients with these diseases also have iron overload.

How is hemochromatosis treated?

Diet changes and other treatments can help ease the symptoms of hemochromatosis. They can also help prevent or delay further damage to your organs:

- **Changes to your diet:** Your healthcare provider will probably ask you to avoid supplements with iron. You may also need to stay away from foods with too much iron and limit vitamin C. Limit your alcohol consumption, too, because it's not good for your liver.

- **Iron chelation therapy:** This medication removes extra iron from your body. It's taken by mouth at home or injected into the blood by a healthcare provider.

- **Therapeutic phlebotomy:** phlebotomy, which means removing blood the same way it is drawn from donors at blood banks. Depending on how severe the iron overload is, a pint of blood will be taken once or twice a week for several months to a year, and occasionally longer. The goal is to bring the iron levels in the blood to well within the normal range and keep them there. Once iron levels return to normal, maintenance therapy, which involves giving a pint of blood every 2 to 4 months for life, begins. Some people may need it more often. An annual blood test will help determine how often blood should be removed.

If another condition caused hemochromatosis, you may need treatment for that, too. And healthcare providers may recommend treating any problems caused by hemochromatosis.

Who is at risk for hemochromatosis?

Immediate relatives of people with hemochromatosis should have their blood tested to see if they have the disease or are carriers, this includes parents, siblings and children.

Doctors should consider testing people who have joint disease, severe and continuing fatigue, heart disease, elevated liver enzymes, impotence, and diabetes, because these conditions may result from hemochromatosis.

People of Northern European descent are more prone to hemochromatosis than are people of other ethnic backgrounds. Men are five times as likely as women are to develop the condition, and they usually experience symptoms at an earlier age.

What is the outlook with hemochromatosis?

The outlook for hemochromatosis depends on the timing of diagnosis and treatment. If not caught and addressed early, severe hemochromatosis can cause serious problems. These complications can include organ damage and possible death.

But hemochromatosis is also a manageable disease. With early detection and treatment, you can survive and live a normal, healthy life. Sometimes organ damage can even be reversed.

Questions to Ask Your Doctor

- What are my iron levels at this time? (Will iron studies be drawn?)

- What is my platelet count?

- What kind of routine lab schedule should I anticipate?

- How often will I need to come in for phlebotomy (blood draw to reduce amount of iron in my bloodstream)?

- Do other members in my family need to be tested?

- Which over the counter medications for pain relief are OK for me to take?

- Should I stop taking vitamin supplements with iron and iodine?

- Are there foods I should be avoiding which naturally have an excess of iron?

- Do I have liver damage?

- Will I need a liver transplant?

- How long will I need treatment?

Hemochromatosis diet

Hemochromatosis causes the body to absorb too much iron from foods. By modifying their diet in specific ways, people with hemochromatosis can minimize the symptoms and reduce the risk of complications.

Most people absorb and lose about 1 milligram (mg) of iron per day. People with hemochromatosis can absorb up to 4 mg of iron each day.

An excessive buildup of iron in the organs can be toxic and cause damage. However, it is possible to maintain healthy iron levels through dietary changes.

Dietary factors

The goal of treating hemochromatosis is to reduce the amount of iron in the body to normal levels.

As well as eating only foods that are low in iron, there are other factors to consider. For example, some dietary components affect how much iron the body absorbs.

Examples include:

- Iron type: Heme iron is easier for the body to absorb than nonheme iron. Plant-based foods contain only nonheme iron, whereas meat, poultry, fish, and seafood contain both heme and nonheme iron.

- Vitamin C: This vitamin enhances nonheme iron absorption.

- Calcium: This mineral can reduce iron absorption.

- Phytates, tannins, and polyphenols: These dietary components limit the absorption of nonheme iron.

What to eat

There are no formal dietary guidelines for people with hemochromatosis, but some foods that may be beneficial include:

Fruits and vegetables

Fruits and vegetables are an important part of any healthful diet. They are rich in vitamins and minerals that are vital for the body to function properly.

Some fruits and vegetables, including spinach, mushrooms, and olives, are high in nonheme iron. As nonheme iron is harder for the body to absorb, they are unlikely to affect iron levels significantly.

People with hemochromatosis have higher levels of oxidative stress that can be damaging. Eating foods that contain antioxidants can counteract the oxidation and protect the cells from damage.

Many fruits and vegetables are high in antioxidants, such as vitamin E and selenium.

Plants also contain phytochemicals or plant compounds that provide protective properties. Examples of phytochemicals include:

- lutein in dark leafy greens

- lycopene in tomatoes

- anthocyanins in beets and blueberries

Lean protein

Lean protein is an essential part of a healthful, balanced diet, but many sources of lean protein contain iron.

Although there is no need for people with hemochromatosis to avoid animal protein completely, it is best to choose animal proteins that contain lower amounts of iron, such as fish and chicken, over iron-rich animal proteins, such as red meat.

Grains, beans, nuts, and seeds

All grains, legumes, seeds, and nuts contain phytic acid, or phytate, which reduces iron absorption.

Eating foods high in phytates, such as beans, nuts, and whole grains, reduces the absorption of nonheme iron from plant foods. As a result, it may reduce total iron levels in the body.

Tea and coffee

Tea and coffee contain tannins, which are types of polyphenol plant compounds.

The tannins in tea and coffee may reduce iron absorption. Drinking these beverages is another way for people with hemochromatosis to manage their iron levels.

Calcium-rich foods

Calcium can inhibit the absorption of both nonheme and heme iron.

Examples of calcium-rich foods include:

- yogurt

- milk

- cheese

- tofu

- green leafy vegetables, such as broccoli

Eggs

Research also suggests that eggs can help inhibit iron absorption.

Eggs contain a protein called phosvitin that binds to iron and prevents absorption.

What to avoid

Doctors generally advise people with hemochromatosis to avoid iron-fortified foods and supplements. Other foods to consider avoiding include:

Red meat

Most red meats, including beef, lamb, and venison, are a rich source of heme iron. Chicken and pork contain lower amounts of heme.

As heme iron is easy for the body to absorb, people with hemochromatosis may wish to avoid most red meat.

Red meat also enhances nonheme iron absorption.

Pairing red meat with foods that reduce iron absorption might also help control iron levels.

Raw shellfish

Shellfish, such as mussels, oysters, and clams, sometimes contain Vibrio vulnificus bacteria.

These bacteria can cause a serious infection called vibriosis.

People with hemochromatosis are more susceptible to vibriosis infection. Therefore, it is important to cook any shellfish thoroughly to kill the bacteria. People can also reduce their risk of infection by discarding any raw shellfish that have open shells and avoiding eating any shellfish that remain unopened after cooking.

Vitamin C

Vitamin C increases the absorption of nonheme iron. Due to this, people with hemochromatosis should avoid vitamin C supplements.

The amount of vitamin C in fruits and vegetables is generally too low to have a significant effect on iron absorption. These foods also contain a variety of other nutrients that are important in a healthful diet.

However, eating foods or drinking beverages high in vitamin C alongside iron-rich foods may enhance iron absorption. For this reason, pairing iron-rich foods with vitamin C-rich foods may not be the best choice for those with hemochromatosis.

People should speak with a doctor to find out how much vitamin C they should be consuming each day.

Fortified foods

Fortified and enriched foods contain added vitamins and minerals to improve nutrition. Many cereal products are fortified with calcium, vitamin D, and iron.

People with hemochromatosis should avoid iron-fortified foods.

Alcohol

Digesting alcohol causes the body to produce substances that damage the liver.

Combining iron and alcohol can increase oxidative stress. This oxidative stress may worsen the effect of hemochromatosis on the body. Alcohol also increases the body's iron stores.

A doctor may suggest to a person with hemochromatosis that they limit their alcohol intake.

HEMOCHROMATOSIS DIET RECIPES

In this part are recipes to keep your hemochromatosis at bay.

Buttermilk Green Tea Roasted

Roasted Chicken

Preparation time

3 hours

INGREDIENTS

- 1 teaspoon dried thyme

- 1 teaspoon dried sage

- 1 teaspoon ground mustard seeds

- 1 tablespoon (2 g) dried rosemary

- 2 teaspoons (10 g) salt

- 1 teaspoon ground black pepper

- 2 tablespoons (30 ml) honey

- 1 cup (240 ml) buttermilk

- 1 cup (240 ml) brewed green tea chilled

- 2 pounds (900 g) skin-on, bone-in chicken pieces (breasts, legs, and so on)

INSTRUCTIONS

1. In a medium bowl, mix together the thyme, sage, mustard seeds, rosemary, salt, and pepper.

2. Stir in the honey, buttermilk, and green tea.

3. Place the chicken and the marinade in a large resealable bag or lidded bowl then refrigerate for at least 2 hours and up to 24 hours.

4. Preheat the oven to 425°F (220°C).

5. Line a medium roasting tray with foil.

6. Let the excess marinade drip off the chicken pieces and place the pieces on the prepared roasting tray.

7. Bake for approximately 30 minutes, until the chicken skin is crispy and the meat reaches an internal temperature of 165°F (74°C).

Blueberry Salad with Grilled Tumeric Chicken

Preparation time

20 minutes

INGREDIENTS

• 1 pound (450 g) chicken breasts, cut into 1-inch (2.5-cm) thick strips

• Salt and black pepper as needed

• 1 teaspoon ground turmeric

• ½ teaspoon curry powder

• 5 tablespoons (75 ml) olive oil, divided

• 4 cups (120 g) coarsely chopped butterhead lettuce

- 1 cup (144 g) fresh blueberries

- ½ cup (60 g) pecan halves

- 2 ounces (58 g) feta or blue cheese, crumbled

INSTRUCTIONS

1. Season the chicken with the salt and pepper.

2. In a small bowl, make a paste with the turmeric, curry powder, and 1 tablespoon (15 ml) of the oil.

3. Coat the chicken strips in the paste and set them aside.

4. Preheat the grill, electric grill, or stovetop grill pan to medium-high heat (400°F [200°C]).

5. Spray it with cooking spray then add the chicken and cook 5 to 7 minutes per side (or 5 to 7 minutes total with a two-sided electric grill) until the chicken reaches an internal temperature of 165°F (74°C).

6. Fill 4 salad bowls with the lettuce and coat it with the remaining 4 tablespoons (60 ml) oil, then top with the chicken strips, blueberries, pecans, and cheese.

Vegetable Quiche

Preparation time

55 minutes

Ingredients

- 1 tbsp. olive oil

- 1/2 cup green onion, chopped

- 1/2 cup onion, chopped

- 1/2 cup zucchini, chopped

- 1 cup spinach

- 3 eggs, beaten

- 1/2 cup milk

- 1 1/2 cups shredded cheese

- 1 deep dish pie crust, precooked

Instructions

1. Preheat the oven to 350°F (177°C).

2. In a large skillet, heat the olive oil.

3. Add the green onion, onion, and zucchini.

4. Cook for 5 minutes.

5. Add the spinach. Cook for an additional 2 minutes. Remove the cooked vegetables from the skillet and set aside.

6. In a mixing bowl, whisk the eggs, milk, half of the cheese, and salt and pepper to taste.

7. Pour the egg mixture into the pie crust. Top with the remainder of the shredded cheese.

8. Bake for 40–45 minutes, or until the eggs are cooked throughout.

Turkey Chili

Preparation time

40 minutes

Ingredients

- 1 tbsp. olive oil

- 1 lb. ground turkey

- 1 large onion, chopped

- 2 cups chicken broth

- 1 (28-ounce) can red tomatoes, crushed

- 1 (16-ounce) can kidney beans, drained and rinsed

- 2 tbsp. chili powder

- 1 tbsp. garlic, chopped

- 1/2 tsp. each cayenne, paprika, dried oregano, cumin, salt, and pepper

Instructions

1. In a large pot over medium heat, heat olive oil.

2. Add the ground turkey and cook until browned.

3. Add the chopped onion and cook until tender.

4. Add the chicken broth, tomatoes, and kidney beans.

5. Add remaining ingredients and stir thoroughly.

6. Bring to a boil then reduce heat to low.

7. Cover and simmer for 30 minutes.

Argentine Diet Merenguitos

Preparation time

2 hours

Ingredients

- 3 egg whites

- 100 grs of diet sugar

Instructions

1. First, put the 3 egg whites and the hundred grams of sugar into a bowl, and mix them with a spoon.

2. Then whip them until they turn into a soft cream.

3. After that, with a pipping bag, make little "snowball" with a little peak in the middle. You should do this in the oven fountain already, so you don't have to move the "snowballs" later (it's a very soft cream so they could fall appart).

4. If you don't have a pipping bag, you can throw the cream with a spoon, this will make the effect of a little peak in the middle too (the only difference will be that it would be smooth).

5. After doing this (there will be about 24 "merenguitos"), turn on the oven in a minimum temperature. If your minimum temp. is too high, open a little bit the oven door. It's very important this, because the "merenguitos" should be white, but still be dry in the interior. That's why it takes about 60 to 90 minutes to cook them.

6. After cooking them, you'll have to wait until they're cold.

7. These are great to eat them alone with coffee or tea. Or exquisite to eat them with cream or "Dulce de Leche" as a dessert.

Glady Chicken veggie mix

Preparation time

15 minutes

Ingredients

- 1 lb Chicken Thigh

- 1 Can of Dark Kidney Beans

- 1/2 cup of Orange (or any color) Bell Pepper

- 1 1/2 cup of Yellow Sweet Corn, Frozen

- 1 tsp of Colgin Natural Hickory Liquid Smoke

- Granulated Garlic to taste

- Granulated Onion to taste

- Pepper to taste

- Salt to taste

Instructions

1. Cut up chicken thighs and cook on stove top using cooking oil spray.

2. Once chicken is partially cooked (about 9 - 10 minutes) add remaining ingredients.

3. Continue cooking until chicken is fully cooked.

Mac and Cheese in Power Pressure Cooker

Preparation time

20 minutes

Ingredients

- 4 serving Broth, chicken: College Inn, Light & Fat Free, 50% less Sodium, Chicken Broth, 1 cup/serv

- 16 oz box of dry: (6 cup cups cooked) Great Value Penne Pasta - Whole Wheat

- 2 tbsp Butter, unsalted

- .75 cup Milk, 2%, with added nonfat milk solids, without added vit A

- 1.75 cup *Kraft Natural Cheese Fat Free Shredded Cheddar

Instructions

1. Add 2 TBS of butter to power pot. Turn on Browning setting. Add 4 cups broth or water, until it comes to a boil. Cancel brown setting.

2. Add 1# (16 oz) uncooked whole wheat pasta. Cover pot with lid and seal. Shut off steam valve. Set power cooker for 5". Then allow to steam for 5 minutes.

3. Remove lid. Add 1/2 cup to 3/4 cup milk. Stir. Add 1: 7 Oz pkg of shredded fat free Cheddar. Stir. Allow to sit on "keep warm " until served, or transfer to serving casserole.

4. Store left overs in refrigerator or freeze. Can reheat serving in micRowave.

Gradly Black Beans and Rice

Preparation time

10 minutes

Ingredients

- 1 1/2 cups of Brown Rice

- One can of Seasoned Black Beans

- 3 tbsp of coconut cream

Instructions

1. Warm black beans and add cocnut cream.

2. Add precooked brown rice until warm.

3. 1/2 a cup makes a Serving

Macaroni, Cheese and Broccoli Quesadilla

Preparation time

15 minutes

Ingredients

- 2 serving Tortillas, MISSION, flour tortilla, 8 inch, 49g

- 1 Serving (makes about 1 cup pre Kraft Macaroni and Cheese Dinner (as prepared, 1c)

- 1 cup Broccoli - chopped - frozen : chop further

- 0.5 cup Kraft Mozzarella, Fat Free

- Butter spray

Instructions

1. Place tortillas on a work surface. On half of each tortilla, evenly distribute macaroni and cheese, broccoli, and mozzarella.

2. In a large skillet or griddle over medium heat, [melt 1/2 table spoon butter] / or, I used ICBINB spray.

3. Place one tortilla, toppings side up, in skillet and cook 1 minute, or until cheese begins to melt.

4. Using a spatula, fold tortilla in half and cook 1 to 2 additional minutes, or until golden and cheese is melted.

5. Flip and cook an additional 30 seconds, or until golden brown.

6. Repeat with remaining tortillas.

7. Slice each tortilla in half and serve immediately.

Gradly Banana But Muffins (With Almond Milk)

Preparation time

30 minutes

Ingredients

• One box of Betty Crocker Banana Nut Muffin Mix

• 1 Cup of Pure Silk Almond Vanilla Milk

• 2 Medium sized Eggs

• 1/4 cup of Vegetable Oil

Instructions

1. Prepapr cups cake based on box insturctions.

2. Makes 12 muffins.

Sixty's Vanilla Trivia Iced Decaf Coffee

Preparation time

3 minutes

Ingredients

• 1.25 cup (8 fl oz) Decaffeinated Coffee = 10 oz

• 4 oz Almond Breeze Almond Milk, Unsweetened Vanilla

• .25 tsp Vanilla Extract

• 1 serving Truvia Natural Sweetener

Instructions

1. Mix in a salsa jar a day in advance.

2. Refrigerate overnight.

3. Stir or shake well before drinking.

4. Can add crushed or cubed ice to The jar Before drinking, or poor over a glass of ice.

Gradly Pesto Pasta

Preparation time

20 minutes

Ingredients

- One Jar of Kroger Basil Pesto (Private Selection)

- One box of Barilla Plus Whole Grain spaghetti (14 oz)

Instructions

1. Cook pasta per box instructions then add pesto

Gradly Roasted Tomatoes and Broccoli Pasta

Preparation time

30 minutes

Ingredients

- 20 plum tomatoes, halved

- 4 tablespoons olive oil

- 1 1/2 tablespoons balsamic vinegar

- 2 large garlic cloves, minced

- 2 teaspoons sugar

- 1 1/2 teaspoons salt

- 1/2 teaspoon freshly ground black pepper

- 1 lb Bow Tie pasta (1 box)

- 12 oz Broccoli, frozen

Instructions

For Tomatoes:

1. Preheat the oven to 425 degrees F.

2. Arrange the tomatoes in a pie pan, cut sides down, in a single layer. Drizzle with olive oil and balsamic vinegar. Sprinkle the garlic, sugar, salt, and pepper over the tomatoes. Roast for 20 minutes.

For Pasta and Broccoli

1. Cook both broccoli and pasta; cook as per instructions on packaging.

2. Combining Ingredients:

3. Once done mix pasta, broccoli, and tomatoes
(with sauce).

Gladly Green Curry w/Turkey

Preparation time

1 hour 10 minutes

Ingredients

• 2 cans of Bright Green Curry Sauce (One Can - 14 oz)

• 4 Cups of Fresh Green Beans (snap)

• 1 Large Sliced Eggplant, fresh

• 1 Fresh ly Sliced/Chopped Yellow Pepper

• 1 1/2 pounds of Chopped Turkey Breast

• 1 cup of Water

Instructions

1) Cook green beans and eggplant over medium heat for 45 mins in one cup of water.

2) In a seperate pan cook turkey meat along with yellow pepper.

3) Drain green beans and eggplant.

4) Heat up green curry sauce in the pot that you used to cook the green beans and eggplant.

5) Once sauce has been heated up add the green beans, eggplant, yellow peppers, and turkey.

Slow Cooker BBQ Shredded Pork Loin

Preparation time

8 hours

Ingredients

- 32 oz Pork, fresh, loin, sirloin (roasts), boneless, separable lean only, cooked, roasted [2 #]

- 16 tbsp BBQ Sauce (Kraft) Orig. [1 cup]

- 16 tbsp GREAT VALUE ALL NATURAL MILD CHUNKY SALSA , no added sugar. [1 cup]

- Cooking Spray

Instructions

1. Spray crockpot base with cooking spray. To make clean up even easier, line pot with cooking bag.

2. Mix BBQ Sauce and Salsa in base. Stir together. Salsa adds spicy flavor.

3. There were 2 loins in package purchased at Walmart. Placed in sauce. Turned to coat.

4. Cook on high 2 hours, then low for 4-6 hours. [or high for 5 hours].

5. Shred meat with 2 forks.

6. I used slotted spoon to serve. Left over Sauce can be stored in refrigerator in glass jar.

Options To Serve:

1. Serve on small bun, or in tortilla, or a lettuce wrap with slaw.

2. I ate in bowl with tomato slices.

To Freeze:

1. Line a cupcake tray with 12 pieces of foil.

2. Spoon BBQ into each.

3. Freeze the tray several hours.

4. Remove individual servings & place In sealable Bag, return to freezer for future meals.

5. Label should include "use by" date.

Gradly Vanilla Ice cream

Preparation time

40 minutes

Ingredients

• Granulated Sugar, 1/4 cup

• Vanilla Extract, 2 tsp

• Lactaid Fat Free Milk, 1 cup

• Heavy Whipping Cream, 16 fl oz

Instructions

1. Combine ingredients and mix well. Make sure that the ingredients are chilled.

2. Turn on ice cream maker and pour in ingredients.

3. All to mix for 20 to 30 minutes depending on desired thickness.

Overnight Vanilla Almond Chia Seed Pudding

Preparation time

10 minutes

Ingredients

- .5 cup Silk Pure Almond Milk - Unsweetened Vanilla Almond Milk

- 1 tsp Vanilla Extract

- .25 cup (8 fl oz) Water, tap — or whey.

- 1 serving Truvia Natural Sweetener

- 38 gram Chia Seed - Spectrum Organic Essentials (1T/12g)

Instructions

1. In any glass container with a tight seal lid, add ingredients in the following order: milk, vanilla, sweetener, and chia seeds. If you would like to add toppings in the morning, use bigger jars, otherwise use smaller jars.

2. Stir well with a spoon or fork, let sit for 1 to 10 minute and stir again. This will prevent lumps. Then refrigerate overnight.

3. When ready to eat, stir well and top with favourite toppings: nuts, berries, fruit, coconut flakes etc.

Store: Refrigerate for up to 5 days.

Gradly Spinach Enchiladas

Preparation time

45 minutes

Ingredients

- Casa Fiesta Enchilada Sauce Mild Mix, 10 oz

- Spinach, fresh, 2 cups

- Cheddar Cheese, 70 grams

- Light Sour Cream, 1/4 cup

- Corn, Raw, 2 cups

- Black Benas, 1 1/2Cups

- Scallions, Raw, 1/4 cup

- 12 Corn Tortillas (approx 6" dia)

Instructions

1. Dip the corn tortilla in the enchilada sauce.

2. Then spoon sour cream, scallions, cheddar cheese, and place spinach on the toritlla.

3. Then roll the tortillas and place in a baking dish.

4. Or layer 6 tortillas at the bottom of a baking dish and then placing spinach, corn, black benas, sour cream, and scallions on top then place 6 tortillas on top.

Gradly Vegetable Coconut Rice

Preparation time

40 minutes

- Ingredients

- 10 oz Peas and carrots, frozen

- 6 cups Deluxe Stir-Fry

- 1 tsp Red Curry Paste

- .5 tbsp Peanut Butter, smooth style

- 4 tbsp Fresh Cilantro

- 13.5 oz Thai Organic Lit Cocnut Milk

- 6 cups Uncle Ben's Paraboiled White Rice

- Salt and Pepper to taste

Instructions

1. Cook rice as per bag/box instructions.

2. Mix currypaste, Peanut Butter and coconut milk together

3. In nonstick wok stirfry cooked rice & frozen vegs

4. Stir in curry sauce

5. When hot stir in chopped cilantro

6. Pour enchilada sauce on top

7. Once all tortillas have been rolled, placed baking dish in the oven at 350 degrees for 35 minutes.

Overnight Chia Flax Pudding with Cherries

Preparation time

5 minutes

Ingredients

• 2 tbsp Flax Seed - Hodgson Mill Milled Flax Seed

• 2 tbsp Seeds Chia Better Body Organic

• 4 oz Almond Breeze Almond Milk, Unsweetened Vanilla

• 4 oz Fage 0% Nonfat Plain Greek Yogurt

• 1 tsp Cinnamon, ground

- .67 cup Great Value Dark Sweet Cherries, pitted & frozen (by DINOSGIRL7779)

- 1 tsp Vanilla Extract

- 1 serving Truvia Natural Sweetener (1 packet)

- .25 tbsp Cocoa powder - Hershey's Special Dark

Instructions

1. Mix all ingredients together

2. Refrigerate at least 4 hours or overnight(optional)

Gradly Low Fat Vanilla Ice cream

Preparation time

30 minutes

Ingredients

- 1 cup Lactaid Fat Free Milk

- 3/4 cup Granulated Sugar

- 2 cups Half and Half Cream

- 2 tsp Vanilla Extract

Instructions

1. Combine ingredients into well mixed and make sure that the ingredients are chilled.

2. Turn on ice cream maker and pour in ingredients.

3. All to mix for 20 to 40 minutes depending on desired thickness.

Gradly Quickly Pasta

Preparation time

12 minutes

Ingredients

- 8 oz Barilla PLUS Thin Spaghetti

- 3/4 cups Yellow Sweet Corn, Frozen

- 3/4 cups Peas, frozen

- 2 cups Spinach, fresh

- 1 tsp Garlic

- 1/2 cup Pacific Natural Foods Organic Beef Broth

- 2 tbsp Olive Oil

- 1 tbsp Thyme, fresh

- 1 tbsp Rosemary

- 1/2 cup Sun Dried Tomatoes

- 6 oz Mozzarella

Instructions

1. Bring water to a biol and cookl pasta as per instructions on the package.

2. Heat olive oil.

3. Once oil has been heated add the frozen corn, sun dried tomatoes, and garlic. Cook this way for 3 minutes.

4. Add in spinach, thyme, rosemary, and broth. Cook for 3 minutes.

5. Drain pasta and mix the pasta in a bowl with the other ingredients.

6. Now add mozzarella

Pumpkin Kodiak Waffle

Preparation time

10 minutes

Ingredients

- 2.67 oz Almond Breeze Almond Milk, Unsweetened Vanilla

- 1 serving Pumpkin-Libby's 100% Pure Pumpkin (1/2 cup)

- 1 serving Beneprotein - 1 scoop or 1 1/2 Tbsp (by POODLEEMOM)

- 26.3 gram kodiak cake buttermilk protein packed

- 1 tsp Pumpkin Pie spice

- 2 serving Egg white, large

Instructions

1. Place ingredients in 2 cup glass measure in order listed. Points come from Kodiak mix (make sure you buy one listed.) This mixes very easily.

2. Preheat the waffle iron, then spray with PAM before adding the mixture.

3. Mine barely covered the entire square waffle maker.

4. I spray the finished waffle with "I can't Believe It's Not Butter " and then frozen blueberries that a put in microwave a minute or two. The blueberries make their own sauce and are zero points.

5. Add everything together: still 2 Smart Points.

Gradly Creamy Grits

Preparation time

55 minutes

Ingredients

- 6 cups water

- 1 1/2 teaspoons salt

- 1 1/2 cups quick cooking or old-fashioned grits
(not instant)

- 2 cups milk

- 1 cup Coffee-Mate Fat Free Original

- 1/2 teaspoon fresh cracked black pepper

- 2 tablespoons Garlic Powder

- 2 tablespoons fresh chopped chives

- One cup equals one serving.

Instructions

1. In a large, heavy saucepan bring the water to a boil.

2. Add salt and grits to boiling water.

3. Stir with a wooden spoon to combine.

4. When the grits thicken, add the milk and whipping cream.

5. Reduce the heat to a simmer, cover the saucepan and cook for 45 minutes to 1 hour, or until the grits are tender, smooth and creamy.

6. Taste and season the grits with the pepper, garlic, and chopped chives.

7. Keep covered and warm until ready to use.

Note:

If the grits seem too runny simply allow to cook a bit longer, uncovered and stirring frequently, until the desired consistency is reached.

Mexican Shrimp Cocktail

Preparation time

15 minutes

Ingredients

- 180 grams Shrimp, cooked (about 5 each serving)

- .5 tsp Baking Soda

- 1 dash Salt

- 2 tbsp Lime Juice, juice of 1 lime

- .5 cup, chopped Onions, raw

- 6 tbsp Pace Chunky Salsa - Mild

- 1 tbsp Ketchup, Heinz

- 50 grams Cilantro, raw

- .5 fl oz Orange Juice

- 1 serving Hass Avocado Fresh (1/2 of Avocado)

- 1 pepper Jalapeno Peppers

- 1 stalk, small (5" long) Celery, raw

- 0.5 cup slices Cucumber (with peel)

Instructions

1. In large bowl, toss thawed shrimp with 1 tsp of salt and the baking soda.

2. Place in refrigerator for 15".

3. Meanwhile, in medium bowl, stir together lime juice with onion, diced cucumber, tomato

product (salsa or puree)., ketchup, cilantro, orange juice, and jalapeño (if using).

4. In a medium pot, cook shrimp if not already cooked.

5. Drain shrimp and rinse under cold running water.

6. If shrimp are large, you may want to dice into bite sized pieces.

7. Place half of shrimp and half of diced avocado in each glass.

8. Cover with remaining ingredients.

9. Garnish with lemon slice and cucumber slice, and cilantro.

Gradly's Mexi-call Chicken

Preparation time

25 minutes

Ingredients

- Frozen Yellow Sweet Corn, 2 cups

- Sliced Mushrooms, fresh, 10 oz

- Black Beans, One Can (drained and rinsed)

- 3 Scallions, Chopped

- Fresh Cilantro Chopped, 4 tbsp

- Pre-Cooked Chicken Breast Chopped, 10 ounces

• Chicken Broth, 1/2 cup

• Light Sour Cream, 1 tbsp (optional)

Instructions

1. Place frozen corn and mushrooms in a lightly oil pan and cook until mushrooms are tender

2. Pour in chicken broth

3. Add in black beans, pre-cooked chicken breast, scallions, and cilantro, stir for 5 minutes.

4. Dish and place sour cream on top (optional)

Gradly Orange Chicken Teriyaki Rice

Preparation time

15 minutes

Ingredients

• 3 Previously Italian Breaded Baked Chicken Breast Fillets

• 1 Package of Frozen Peas and Carrots

• 2 Oranges (sliced or diced)

• 1 1/2 Cup Brown Rice

• 1 tbsp Teriyaki Sauce

• 1 tbsp Extra Light Olive Oil

Instructions

1. Combine all ingredients in a pan until warm.

Gradly Fruit Topping

Preparation time

5 minutes

Ingredients

- 6 Large Strawberries (Sliced)

- 20 Blueberries

- 1/4 Cup Fat Free Cool Whip

Instructions

1. Slice strawberries.

2. Mix all ingredients into a a bowl.

3. 1/4 cup equals a serving

Easy Granola

Preparation time

40 minutes

Ingredients

- Local Honey, 0.5 cup

- Canola Oil, 2 tbsp

- Salt, 1 tsp

- Oats_100% Whole Grain_Old Fashioned_uncooked, 4 cup

- Almonds, .5 cup, sliced (remove)

- Cashew Nuts, dry roasted, .5 cup, halves and whole

- Walnuts, .5 cup, chopped

- Dried Cranberries, 0.33 cup, chopped

- Raisins, .33 cup, packed

- Sunflower Seeds, with salt added, .33 cup

Instructions

1. Preheat oven to 350 degrees.

2. Measure honey, salt, and canola in a Pyrex cup; heat in microwave for 10 seconds twice.

3. Measure remaining ingredients except fruit and seeds into 1 or 2 (9x11) baking dishes, lined with parchment.

4. Stir. Pour warm honey mixture over the dry ingredients. Stir. Bake for 30 minutes, stirring every 10 to 15 minutes.

5. Meanwhile, lightly toast the seeds in a dry non-stick pan. Do not add until the last ten minutes to the granola mix in the oven.

6. Add the dry fruit after finished baking.

7. Mix well. Cool.

Marta Stewart's Chocolate Custard Cup

Preparation time

55 minutes

Ingredients

- 1 1/2 cups half-and-half

- 1 teaspoon pure vanilla extract

- 3 large egg yolks

- 1/4 cup sugar

- Pinch of salt

- 3 ounces unsweetened baking chocolate squares

Instructions

Preheat oven to 325 degrees.

Bring a kettle of water to a boil or heat in 4 cup Pyrex pitcher in microwave.

 In a medium saucepan, bring half-and-half and vanilla just to a boil.

Remove from heat.

Add chopped chocolate and stir until melted and smooth.

Place egg yolks, sugar, and salt in a medium bowl. Beat until light.

Whisking constantly, gradually add hot half-and-half mixture.

Skim any foam from surface. (I didn't have any foam.)

Divide mixture among four (4-6 ounce) custard cups, and place in a baking dish just large enough to hold them.

Place in oven, and pour enough boiling water in dish to come halfway up sides of cups.

 Drape a sheet of aluminum foil over top of baking dish (do not seal).

Bake custards until just set but still slightly wobbly, 40 to 45 minutes.

Remove cups from dish;

Refrigerate until chilled, at least 2 hours.

Chocolate Custard

Ingredients

• 1 cup Land O Lakes® Heavy Whipping Cream

• 1/3 cup milk

• 6 ounces high-quality semi-sweet chocolate, chopped

• 4 Land O Lakes® All-Natural Egg yolks

Instructions

1. Place cream and milk in heavy 2-quart saucepan.

2. Cook over medium-high heat 2-3 minutes, stirring occasionally, until mixture just comes to a boil.

3. Immediately remove from heat.

4. Add chocolate; whisk until melted and smooth.

5. Whisk yolks in bowl just to blend.

6. Gradually whisk warm chocolate mixture into beaten yolks.

7. Return chocolate mixture to same saucepan.

8. Cook over medium heat 8-10 minutes, stirring constantly, until mixture thickens and just begins to bubble. Do not boil.

Fudge Brownies/ Whole wheat

Preparation time

35 minutes

Ingredients

- ¾ cup sugar

- ½ cup whole wheat flour

- ¼ cup unsweetened cocoa powder

- ½ teaspoon salt

- ¼ teaspoon baking powder

- 1 stick (1/2 cup) melted butter, plus a little extra for greasing (I used Parkay)

- 2 eggs

- 1 teaspoon vanilla extract

- ¾ cup chocolate chips

Instructions

1. Preheat the oven to 350 degrees F. Generously grease a 8X8 or 9X9 square baking dish with a little melted butter (a pastry brush makes this job super easy).

2. In a large mixing bowl whisk together the sugar, flour, cocoa powder, salt, and baking powder.

3. Make a well (hole) in the center and drop in the butter, eggs, and vanilla extract.

4. Mix together thoroughly and then fold in the chocolate chips with a rubber spatula.

5. Add the brownie batter to the baking dish and use the spatula to flatten out the top into one even layer.

6. Bake for about 30 minutes and let cool before slicing into squares.

Quick Lentil Sauce and Spaghetti

Preparation time

15 minutes

Ingredients

• Lentils, 1 cup (precooked)

- 1 can Diced Tomatoes with Onions

- 2 servings of Whole Wheat thin Spaghetti (read label on box)

- 2 TBS shredded Parmesan

Instructions

1. Have lentils precooked according to package directions. Can freeze in sandwich bags.

2. Boil pasta according to box directions. Mine takes 6 minutes.

3. Heat diced tomatoes with lentils.

4. Mix tomato lentil sauce with spaghetti. I measure 1/2 cup per person. Usually have leftovers for tomorrow's lunch.

5. Top each serving with 1 TBS shredded Parmesan.

Baked Potato Flake and Fried Chicken Thighs

Preparation time

40 minutes

Ingredients

• egg white, fresh, 1 large (

• Mrs. Dash (R) Garlic & Herb Seasoning Blend, 0.25 tsp or your favorite seasoning

• Chicken Thigh, 200 grams

- *Hungry Jack Mashed Potato flakes, 0.25 cup

Instructions

1. Preheat oven to 425.

2. Wash & dry chicken thighs.

3. Dip to coat all sides in egg white, then dip to coat in dry potato flakes.

4. Put in sprayed 8x8 Pyrex dish.

5. Bake 30 to 35 minutes. I turn pan around half way through to brown more evenly.

Quick Cheesy Salmon Noodle Bake

Preparation time

45 minutes

Ingredients

- Pink Salmon, Chicken of the Sea, skinless/boneless, chunk style in water, 12 oz (remove)

- Velveeta Light Cheese Product, 4 oz (remove)

- Milk, 2%, 0.5 cup (remove)

- Green Peppers (bell peppers), 1 cup, chopped (remove)

- Carrots, raw, 1 carrot (7-1/2") (remove)

- Mushrooms, canned, 0.5 cup (remove)

- *No Yolk Broad Noodles, 4 oz (remove)

Instructions

1. Preheat oven to 375.

2. Start a pot of water to boil.

3. In a small pot, start the milk to heat and add the Velveeta 2%. Turn off before it scalds.

4. Clean, peel, & dice the carrot.

5. Add it to the pot of water as it is getting warm.

6. Clean & dice the bell pepper.

7. Add to the boiling water.

8. When it returns to a boil, add the noodles to the water and boil for half the time. DRAIN.

9. Remove bones & skin from the salmon.

10. Stir & break up in a casserole dish that was sprayed with PAM.

11. Stir in the drained mushroom stems and pieces.

12. When the noodle mixture is finished, stir into the salmon mixture in the casserole.

13. Pour the melted cheese sauce over the noodle mixture & stir well.

14. Place in oven to finish cooking for 20-30"

Maid Rites

Preparation time

30 minutes

Ingredients

- Ground beef, extra lean, 16 oz (remove)

- Celery, raw, 1 cup, diced (remove)

- Onions, raw, 1 cup, chopped (remove)

- *Heinz Worchestershire Sauce, 6 tsp (remove)

- Cider Vinegar, 2 tbsp (remove)

- *Mustard, Ground, 3 tsp (remove)

- Lemon juice, 1 tbsp (remove)

- Brown Sugar, 6 tsp packed (remove)

• Pepper, black, 1 dash (remove)

Instructions

1. Saute the hamburger and pour off grease.

2. Add remaining ingredients & simmer until thick.

3. Suggestions not included in calories:

4. Serve on a bun. Serve with Mac-Salad & cucumber & tomato.

Coachmn's Salad

Preparation time

15 minutes

Ingredients

- Dressing Ingredients:

- Sour Cream, fat free, 1/2 cup

- Reduced Fat Mayonnaise, 1 tbsp

- Cider Vinegar, 1 tbsp

- Splenda, 1 tsp

- Fresh Chives, 5 tbsp chopped

- Salt, 1 dash

- Pepper, black, 1 dash

Salad Ingredients (Cut in size of match sticks).

- Ham, extra lean, (5% fat), 1 cup

- Cucumber (with peel), 1 cucumber (8-1/4") (remove seeds)

- Bell Pepper - Red - 1 large (164 gram)

- Green Beans (snap), 1 cup [fresh, blanched]

- Hard Boiled Egg, 2 large - diced

- Onions, raw, 1 large - slice in thin rings

Instructions

1. Mix dressing ingredients in Pyrex bowl with lid.

2. Add prepped salad ingredients. Mix well.

3. Best if refrigerated overnight before serving.

4. Serving Size: Divide between six serving dishes to find quantity.

Oatmeal, Oatbran, Flax

Preparation time

30 minutes

Ingredients

• Oatmeal, Old Fashion (1/2 C. dry), 4 serving (remove)

• Oat Bran, 0.5 cup (remove)

• Flax, Cold Milled, Ground Golden Flax Seed (2TB=14g), 14 gram (remove)

• Milk, nonfat, 2 cup (remove)

Instructions

1. Mix together.

2. Add cinnamon or pumpkin spice & or vanilla.

3. Cook according to package directions.

Kidney Bean and Taraggon Salad

Preparation time

5 minutes

Ingredients

• Champagne vinegar [I use red wine vinegar]

- Dijon mustard

- Extra-virgin olive oil

- 15-ounce cans red kidney beans, drained and rinsed

- Minced fresh tarragon

- Chopped red onion

- Sea salt and freshly ground back pepper

Measurements for calculations:

- Cider Vinegar, 1 tbsp (remove)

- Grey Poupon Dijon Mustard, 1 tsp (remove)

- Olive Oil, 1 tbsp (remove)

- Beans, red kidney, 1.5 cup (remove)

- Tarragon, ground, 1 tbsp (remove) fresh not in nutrition library
- Onions, raw, 0.5 cup, chopped (remove)

Ingredients

1. Combine the vinegar and mustard in a large bowl.

2. Whisk in the olive oil until emulsified.

3. Add the beans, tarragon and onion.

4. Season with sea salt and pepper to taste, and mix to combine.

Salmon Burger on a Bed of Baby Green

Preparation time

10 minutes

Ingredients

- 1 14.75 oz. can of Wild Alaskan salmon

- 3 scallions, minced

- 1 tablespoon finely grated peeled fresh ginger

- 1 large egg white

- 1 tablespoon soy sauce [light]

- 1 tablespoon olive oil

- 2 cups baby greens

Instructions

1. Drain salmon and then stir together with scallions, and ginger in a large glass or ceramic bowl until well combined.

2. Beat together egg white and soy sauce in a small bowl and stir into salmon mixture; form into 4 (1/2-inch-thick) patties.

3. Heat the olive oil in a 12-inch skillet over medium heat.

4. Add patties and cook, carefully turning once, until golden brown and cooked through, approximately 6 to 7 minutes.

5. Arrange ½ cup of greens per plate.

6. Place hot burgers on the greens, serve immediately.

Stuffed Cabbage

Preparation time

2 hours

Ingredients

- Cabbage, fresh, 1 head, medium (about 5-3/4" dia)

- Ground Chicken, 16 oZ

- Egg white, 1 serving

- Parmesan Cheese, grated, 0.3 cup

- Cauliflower, raw, 1 cup - chopped in fine pieces.

- Mrs. Dash (R) Garlic & Herb Seasoning Blend, 0.25 tsp

- Tomato Paste, 0.065 cup = 1 TBS

- Canned Tomatoes, 1.5 cup

Instructions

1. Boil 8 cups of water in an 8 quart pot.

2. Mix ground chicken, egg & herb blend in mixing bowl.

3. Add 1/3 cup grated Parmesan cheese, raw cauliflower.

4. Remove core of cabbage with tip of knife.

5. Reduce water in pot to medium.

6. Carefully place head of cabbage in boiling water and simmer 4-5 minutes until outer leaves are soft.

7. Remove cabbage from water and peel outer soft leaves until you reach uncooked interior of cabbage.

8. Place leaves on platter and return uncooked cabbage to pot. Boil 4-5 minutes more and repeat procedure above until all cabbage leaves are cooked.

9. Stuff leaves with 1/4 cup to 1/2 cup meat mixture by placing mixture in center of cabbage then folding over bottom, sides and top of cabbage leaf (Note: some leaves are smaller and will require less meat mix).

10. Place stuffed cabbage in Dutch Oven or a roasting pan. Season tomatoes & tomato paste from a tube with Mrs. Dash Herb blend of choice & then puree in pan with blender.

11. Cover stuffed cabbage with pureed tomatoes and bake covered at 350 degrees for 1 1/2 hours.

Dilled Carrot, Cabbage and Parsnip Soup

Preparation time

40 minutes

Ingredients

- Canola Oil, 2 tbsp

- Carrots, raw, 2 cup, chopped

- Cabbage, fresh, 1 cup, chopped

- Parsnips, 0.666 parsnip (9" long)

- Mrs. Dash (R) Original Blend, 0.25 tsp

- 1 Bay Leaf whole - remove before adding to blender.

- Campbell's 25% less salt fat free chicken broth, 0.66 cup & add water to make 2 cups of liquid.

- Dill weed, fresh, 5 sprigs

Instructions

1. Preheat at medium: dutch oven on stove top while prepping veggies.

2. Add chopped veggies and stir in the oil.

3. Cook a couple minutes to soften, not to brown.

4. Add 2 cups of low fat chicken broth [I use homemade so it is low sodium and cooked with herbs]

5. Bring to simmer for about 30-40" until veggies are fork tender.

6. Cool - in refrigerator or in blender container. Do not blend until cool.

7. Blend until smooth.

8. Add sprigs of dill with reheating. [remove stems]

Grated Raw Beet Salad

Preparation time

10 minutes

Ingredients

- Beets, fresh, 227 grams = 1/2 pound

- Orange Juice, 1.5 fl oz = 3 TBS

- Lemon Juice, 0.5 fl oz = 1 TBS

- Olive Oil, 1 tbsp (remove)

- Fresh Chives, 2 tbsp chopped (remove)

- Romaine Lettuce (salad), 4 inner leaf (remove)

• Salt, 1 dash or as desired

Instructions

1. Peel the beets with a vegetable peeler, and grate in a food processor fitted with the shredding blade. [I use a hand grater]

2. Combine the orange juice, lemon juice and olive oil.

3. Toss with the beets and herbs.

4. Season to taste with salt.

5. Line a salad bowl or platter with romaine lettuce leaves, top with the grated beets and serve.

Advance preparation:

The grated beets can be dressed and kept in the refrigerator, covered well, for a couple of days. They become more tender but don't lose their texture, and the mixture becomes even sweeter as the beet juices mingle with the citrus. Toss again before serving.

Tomatoes Avocado Relish (Salsa)

Preparation time

10 minutes

Ingredients

- Lemon juice, 1 tbsp

- Balsamic Vinegar, 1 tbsp

- Olive Oil, 1 1tsp

- Garlic, 1 clove - grated or chop fine

- Onions, raw, 0.5 cup, chopped

- Red Ripe Tomatoes, 1 cup [whole] cherry tomatoes - quartered

- Cilantro, raw, 4 tbsp

- Avocados, California (Haas), 0.5 fruit without skin and seeds

Instructions

1. Mix liquid ingredients in medium bowl or serving dish.

2. Add each of the following ingredients and stir with each addition.

3. Cover and refrigerate 30 minutes to overnight before serving.

Eggplant Stacks

Preparation time

35 minutes

Ingredients

Eggplant, fresh, 1 eggplant, unpeeled (approx 1-1/4 lb

Prego Spaghetti Sauce, 16 tbsp

Sargento Reduced Fat Provalone 4 Slice, cut in quarters

Olive Oil, 3 tbsp

Instructions

1. Preheat oven to 400 degrees.

2. Line baking pan with foil.

3. Spray with PAM.

4. Wash the eggplant.

5. Slice into 16 slices.

6. Brush each side with a minimum of Olive oil.

7. Place 8 of the larger slices of the eggplant in the baking dish. Top each with1 TBS of spaghetti sauce.

8. Then top each with a 1/4 slice of the Provolone.

9. Repeat a layer of eggplant [brushed with oil].

10. Top with 1 tbs of tomato sauce on each.

11. Top each with 1/4 slcie of cheese.

12. Place in oven and bake for 20 to 25 minutes until cheese is bubbly and slightly brown.